SCOTT LAY

Diabetes

The First 7 Days After Diagnosis

This book was professionally typeset on Reedsy.
Find out more at reedsy.com

Contents

1

Introduction

First, let me say that your new journey as someone that has diabetes is not nearly as difficult as you might think. Yes, there are things that are forever going to change in your life, but the benefits of this change far outweigh the consequences of neglecting to manage your disease. Diabetes is a serious illness that can and will have a devastating impact on your quality of life if left untreated. By properly managing your blood sugar, most people will live very productively and avoid many of the health issues that are caused by diabetes. The goal here is not to make you an overnight expert in everything diabetes, but rather to get your mind in the right place so that you can quickly make progress. Watching your blood sugar levels improving is motivating and is the encouragement that you need in the beginning. You will, over time, learn much more about diabetes and how to manage it, what you can and cannot eat and even find yourself getting excited about trying new recipes for some tasty dishes. The overall tone that I want to convey here is that yes, this is a big deal, but for most people it is very manageable and given some time can become "normal." Properly managing your blood sugar will actually improve your life, not make it miserable.

So, for whatever reason you ended up seeing your Doctor and was told you have diabetes. Wow! Now what? This is devastating news. You are too busy to be slowed down with something like this. You have a demanding job that isn't going to allow you to do all the things that are necessary to manage this disease. You have tried diets in the past just because you wanted to lose a little weight and they not only didn't work, it simply put a strain on you lifestyle. If I was asked right now to try to sum up your thoughts and feelings about your current situation, the one word I would use for most people is "aimless." Aimless is a better word than confused or lost because right now you feel like you have to change your whole world and have no idea which direction to even begin walking. You might be scared, or at least a little apprehensive about your future. I would hope that your Doctor or Nurse gave you some solid advice on where to begin but it is hardly enough to answer all the questions that you don't even know you have right now. You definitely know you have a long list of them, but this is a lot to comprehend and at this point, you just know that everything is different now.

There is also the other possibility and the way that I felt when the Doctor came in the room and said, "We have work to do. You are without question a type 2 diabetic and your blood sugar levels are dangerously high." I was relieved. I had felt so bad for so long and I finally had an answer as to why. I can't say I was thrilled with the news, but I knew enough about diabetes to know that getting my blood sugar under control was the key to getting back to a healthier and happier me. I was ready to get started at that very moment and even with all my positivity and enthusiasm, I quickly found myself asking my phone question after question and those questions usually started with the phrase, "how many carbs are in (fill in the blank?)"

As I said before, I was highly motivated, but I knew I had big obstacles in the way. Like many Americans, I had spent most of the last decade without health insurance and even when I did have it, who has time to schedule a doctors appointment? Furthermore, insurance or not, there is still a significant expense involved so to make a long story short, I continued to procrastinate on seeing a doctor. As an over the road truck driver, I convinced myself that my only problem was that I was eating horribly and terribly out of shape. Turns out I was mostly right, but the problem had progressed to a point that forced me to seek help and I was way past ready to do whatever it took to start feeling better. My immediate concern was how was I going to manage eating properly while on the road? I just automatically assumed that there would be no more fast food or any food for that matter that could be found at or near a Truckstop. I was wrong in that assumption and the purpose of this book is to help ease some of your concerns and help you take the first steps on this new path that you find yourself on.

2

Getting Your Thoughts Together

The Plan

It should go without saying that it is imperative that you closely follow the instructions of your healthcare provider. Everyone has different circumstances, and some people have other health issues that may need to be taken into consideration. A diagnosis of diabetes means that your body can not properly regulate your blood sugar levels, therefore this regulation must be accomplished by what you eat. Medications are also used to assist in this process, but these medications are not magic, it is your diet that will determine your success. Too many carbohydrates are the enemy and carbohydrates just happen to be in most of the foods that we all love to eat. Being newly diagnosed with diabetes, it is likely that your blood sugar levels are too high, and you are going to reduce these numbers by dramatically reducing the amount of carbohydrates that you consume. At some point soon, you are going to get these levels closer to the normal range which will require

4

you to not only keep them down, but also not allow them to get too low. This balancing act will be much easier than it may sound because by then you will have a better understanding of how certain foods effect your blood sugar. For now, the plan is to know how many carbs you are consuming in everything that you put in your mouth.

Again, always follow the advice of your doctor but it is recommended that diabetics eat 3 meals per day and the amount of carbs that you consume should be between 45 and 60 grams per meal. Additionally, the recommendation is 2-3 snacks per day between meals that contain between 15 and 20 grams of carbohydrates. In my case, my levels were initially very high, and I did not consume nearly the amount of carbohydrates that these guidelines recommend which for me produced very good results that were evident within two weeks. Not only were my numbers looking better with each passing day, but I noticed a remarkable change in my energy level and began to feel better than I had in several years.

What You Need to Learn Now

I want to once again offer some encouragement here. While learning how many carbs are in every single thing you eat sounds like an impossible task, the good news is that's not necessary. You will gradually begin to become much more familiar with many foods and the amount of carbs they contain. In the beginning, understanding the most common foods we consume as either "good" or "bad" is a great way to get started. You must dramatically reduce or even better, stop eating bread, pasta, potatoes (french fries), rice, and anything that would be considered a desert or "sweets." I'm not saying that you will never again eat any of these foods but once you are successfully managing your blood sugar, some of these foods can be eaten in small quantities on occasions. At some point, you are going to get a craving for something that will not leave you alone. A strategy that seems to work is to have a couple of small bites of whatever is haunting you and treat that as a small reward for all of the "bad" foods that you have been avoiding.

What can you eat? Proteins such as chicken, beef, pork and fish are all good but avoid eating meat or fish that has been breaded and deep fried. The better choice is always baked, grilled or broiled. Fruits and vegetables are good foods, but it is important to begin to learn about the carbohydrates in fruits. Fresh fruit is a great option as part of your daily diet, but it does contain carbohydrates and some fruits are better than others. I encourage you to do some research to find out which ones to eat in moderation. Speaking of fruit, be very careful with juices such as orange juice or grape juice because they are typically high in carbs and should be avoided.

I don't really intend to get very detailed about what to eat or not eat here. My goal is to get you thinking in the right direction. You and your doctor should decide what is the appropriate amount of carbs for you and then you should work hard to meet those goals. It is going to be important going forward that you pay close attention to food labels and how to read them. Hopefully your healthcare provider discussed this with you, but practice is the best teacher. There are some good videos available through internet searches and learning about food labels is imperative. Remember, in the early stages of your journey, serving size and total carbohydrates is what you should be looking at when it comes to labels, and you should be looking at the label of anything you are considering eating.

Start Forming Your New Habits Today

There is not much else to say about this other than maybe a quick review. The plan is to dramatically reduce your carbohydrate intake and we are going to do that by avoiding consuming carbohydrates. You should quickly figure out what foods that you commonly eat must be cut out of your diet and replace them with a good alternative. For at least the first couple of weeks keep your phone handy and ask the question? How many carbs are in grapes? or Bananas? Or whatever? You will find that within a short period of time you will begin to learn what and how much of these foods you can have.

Another very important thing to mention here and possibly one of the more difficult things to adjust to is what you choose to drink. By far, the best choice is always going to be water. For many of us, soft drinks have been a huge part of our diet for much of our lives. Diet drinks are not a great alternative but realistically, they can be helpful during this transition. I encourage you to look for better choices and also want to mention something else while we are on the topic of "diet" drinks. Just because a food or drink is labeled "diet" doesn't necessarily mean that it is low in carbohydrates. Always look at the labels.

3

Building Your Team

The Most Important Player

This one is easy; you are without question the star player on this team. Ultimately it is up to you to manage your blood sugar levels and it is you that is responsible for ensuring that you get and stay as healthy as possible. It is entirely possible that you are in a similar position today that I was at the time of my diagnosis. I was sick and had been for a long time. I want to encourage you to take this very seriously. Within two weeks I noticed that things were starting to change. At a month, I could honestly say that I felt better than I had in literally years. My progress occurred much quicker than I expected, and I sincerely hope that yours does too but any progress is a cause for celebration. As you begin to feel better, everything starts to change. I was struggling to drag myself through each day for a long time and that takes a toll on every aspect of your life. I have dreams again, things I want to accomplish, places I want to go and a life that I want to enjoy. I want this for you too. Take your progress and run with it and if you have setbacks, work through them and do what you can to be as healthy as you can.

Again, everyone has their unique situation which can make this a very different experience for each of us. In my case, I live alone and work alone so my experience could be very different than someone who lives with others. For me, a trip to the grocery store resulted in a cart that only contained things I could eat. This will likely not be the case for someone that is shopping for or living with family members. Given some time, your journey with diabetes might change some of the eating habits of your family for the better. In the early days of navigating this you should expect to eat differently than other members of your household. Understanding this just continues to drive home the point that this is your game to play, and you are the MVP.

Family, Friends, and Your Doctor

We have already touched on family dynamics, but we should expand a little and also talk about other support. Just like you have no idea where to start, your spouse, significant other, children and friends are all in that boat with you. Particularly with close family members, it will be important that they begin to understand and learn about diabetes as you do. In some cases, your family, or people that you are close to might be the person that does the grocery shopping, prepares the meals, or both. In this case, it is very easy to understand that they are playing a key role in your health, and they would have to have the knowledge necessary to help in your success. Family members can assist in any number of ways that might include meal planning, monitoring your blood sugar levels, or maybe just reminding you to take your medication. You are going to want to incorporate some sort of physical activity into your routine and family members may want to join you as you take your walk or go swimming. Emotional support and encouragement from family and friends can be very motivating in helping you stay on the right track. These people care about you and your well-being so keeping them involved and informed about what is going on with your health will be beneficial to everyone.

Your relationship with your doctor and other medical professionals is also a part of building a good team. Many people simply show up for an appointment, briefly answer any questions the doctor or nurse may have, listen to the instructions and leave. Let your doctor know that you are extremely interested in learning what you can do to improve your health. Make notes of any questions that you have since your last visit and be prepared to briefly explain what you have learned about your condition and the steps you are taking to correct it.

Internet, Social Media, and Books

The resources on anything diabetes is abundant across many different platforms on the internet. I would suggest that you use these resources initially to find out what foods are low in carbs so you can begin to eat the things that are going to lower your numbers. You will quickly become familiar with the common foods to avoid such as pasta, bread and potatoes and you will also begin to understand what you can eat. Surprisingly, many of the foods that you have been eating most of your life are still going to be good choices to eat now. For instance, everything that you would put on a typical hamburger is ok to eat except for the bread. Simply build your burger on a plate or in a bowl and grab a fork. Of course, you can't throw a pile of french fries or potato chips next to it, but substitutions are available. You can find some great recipes and ideas on nearly every popular social media platform complete with video instructions on how to prepare them. If you happen to enjoy cooking or preparing food, you will find that there is no possible way to try all the recipes that look so tasty, there simply isn't enough time in day. Social media and the internet is an invaluable resource for not only learning about diabetes but finding creative ways to help manage it.

Another plentiful source of information is found in the form of books. Mountains of books have been written on all aspects of diabetes and a quick internet search can result in a confusing "where do I start?" for the newly diagnosed. Again, this diabetes thing is brand new to you and learning all this new information will come in time. I want to stress the overall purpose of what you are reading now. Our initial goal when first diagnosed is to begin to lower our blood sugar levels and begin the process of learning how to manage them. In other words, we need to drastically reduce our carbohydrate intake now and while our blood sugar levels are improving, we start figuring out how to maintain them once they are at healthy levels. The point being, dive in as deep as you like into learning everything you can about your condition and how to manage it, but don't stress over it. For most of us, a slow progression of learning and building on that knowledge is the most effective approach.

If books are what you are interested in, the internet or a trip to the library will offer ample amounts of books that include everything from technical medical information to day to day tips on managing diabetes. At this early stage, just looking at recipes and meal plans can be helpful by exposing yourself to ideas of how to best change your eating habits. Cookbooks and meal plans, snack hacks, and even desserts, there are books out there for anything you want to know and can be a great resource.

So, to sum this up, everyone's team will look different but what will always be the same is you are the key to this being successful. Some people will have doctors, family, friends and an abundance of help as they move forward. Others may see a doctor every month or two and build their team around people they have never met such as content creators on social media platforms and Authors of books. It doesn't matter what your particular circumstance is, all the help in the world can't keep you from eating half of a cheesecake, it is ultimately up to you to manage your health.

This is a good place to talk about something else that is important to this conversation. It is a well-known fact that eating healthily can be more expensive than eating the foods we are typically accustomed to buying. By using the resources we have previously mentioned, you can develop strategies to make this work within your budget. Again, simple internet searches or books can be very helpful in exposing you to content creators, articles and books that can help you find ways to eat healthy foods without breaking your budget. The most important thing about this is to not allow it to be an excuse for not taking care of yourself. It is only an obstacle that is well worth overcoming

4

What Are You Going to Eat?

he Good News

If you think that you are going to be walking around hungry and chewing celery every day, you are definitely wrong. While learning how to eat a good balanced diet takes time and you want to eventually get to that point, the initial goal is just a few simple things. First, cut out all the obvious foods that are high in carbohydrates like bread, pasta and potatoes. Find low carb alternatives to the high carb drinks that you have likely been consuming for most of your life. Water is the best choice but after a day or two of water only, I found it very difficult to get even close to excited about the thought of a bottle of water. I initially tried to overcome this with unsweet tea and lemon which I like but even that wasn't working. I know that diet soft drinks are controversial and from what I have read these are not great alternatives, but these drinks were very helpful in the first few weeks. I think it is more the familiar fizz of the carbonation that satisfied something in my brain, and it worked for me. I encourage you to eventually do some research and limit your consumption of artificially sweetened foods but remember what we are trying to accomplish. We are taking the huge leap of profoundly reducing our carbohydrate intake while taking the baby steps of changing everything about our eating habits. This is a process, and we will get better at this with each passing day.

If you like all the common proteins like beef, pork, chicken and fish, you will be delighted to know that these are all very much in the column of food you can eat. You will want to avoid eating any of these that have been breaded and fried such as fried chicken or breaded fish, but steak, grilled chicken, pork chops or baked fish are all good options. The big difference in how your meal will now look is what is next to it on the plate. A big scoop of mashed potatoes or a pile of french fries must be replaced with something much lower in carbohydrates. There are countless options for side dishes like a salad, sautéed vegetables, fresh fruit, anything that you like that is a low or no carb choice will complete a good meal. If breakfast is your favorite meal, eggs, bacon or sausage, and fresh fruits are perfect. You will need to stay away from the toast with jelly and the glass of orange juice but it's still a very good and tasty meal. When you start to realize that there are plenty of things that you can eat and lots of creative ways to prepare them, the idea of being on a special diet is no longer a source of stress. All we are doing is reducing the amount of carbohydrates in everything we eat.

My favorite part of a Superbowl party or holiday gathering was always the vegetable tray and I could build one as good as anyone.

- Celery
- Carrots
- Broccoli
- Cauliflower
- Dill Pickles
- Cherry Tomatoes

- Several types of cheese
- Pepperoni
- Hard Salami
- Dip (whatever you like)

Just double check the label on the dip that you choose, and you can have everything on this tray. The only thing I had to remove from my traditional tray was sweet pickles. You will find that many of the foods that you already love are still things you can eat.

Admittedly, snacks and sweets were not much of a challenge for me because it was not a big part of what I ate before my diagnosis. I could tear up a bag of chips and wash them down with a large soft drink, but it wasn't something I did regularly. There are a ton of healthy alternatives to these high carb snacks, and you will find the foods that are both low in carbs and satisfying. You might be surprised to find out how delicious a little peanut butter spread on raw cauliflower can be and it is my go-to snack when I want something sweet. The challenge here is by far the fact that you can't just walk into a convenience store and walk out with a snack when you are hungry. You will find that it takes a little effort and usually the best way to handle this is to bring your snacks with you. Take a small cooler with the things you like to eat with you to work or wherever you may be going that won't have good food choices available. In the beginning you will likely find that you are eating the same few things which is fine, the goal is low carb intake. Over time this will change, and your choices will become more diversified as you learn what you like and more importantly, learn to like things you had no idea you would.

There is no possible way that I can say you should eat, this, this, and that. I have no idea of the kind of foods you like and the things you absolutely cannot eat. Luckily for me, I have always liked almost anything that was food and was never accused of being particularly picky about the food I ate. I'm not telling you exactly what to eat, I'm saying what you eat must have way less carbohydrates than you have been consuming. Cutting the big ones, (bread, pasta, and Potatoes) and consuming no sugary drinks is a huge accomplishment that will produce good results. Combining that with reading food labels and learning about carbs in fruit is the blueprint for reducing your carbohydrate intake which is the key to healthy blood sugar levels.

The Bad News

There isn't any bad news. Yes, you are getting ready to make big changes but hopefully my message is becoming clear. These changes are a bit challenging in the beginning but not really as hard as one might think. By making these changes you are going to feel better, sleep better, breathe better, you will begin to lose a little weight, but the most important thing is what you are doing for your future. Diabetes can and will have devasting consequences on your health if poorly managed or left untreated. By doing the things necessary to successfully manage your diabetes, you are reducing the risk that this disease will increasingly have you sick and/or hospitalized for the rest of your life. If there is any bad news to deliver, I would say that by not taking your diabetes seriously, you can expect to gradually experience a number of medical issues that will impact your quality of life in a negative way.

The Hardest Part

Hydration is important to the health of every living thing on the plant and is particularly important to your health as a diabetic. Finding something to drink that is low in carbohydrates and something that I could drink on a regular basis has been my biggest obstacle. At this point I have found several options that I like, and I have these options during the day. In the warmer months, it is much easier for me to drink water, I actually crave it when the weather is hot. I'm not saying that hydration is the hardest part, what I am saying is it was the hardest part for me. Your hardest part might be something entirely different and what I can say about this is find a way to work through it. Whatever you are having trouble with will get better tomorrow, or next week, or next month. When you do realize that something is a problem, focus on it and work through a way to overcome it.

$$5$$

Thinking Long Term

Take This Slowly

Relax. Take a deep breath. Hopefully what we have talked about so far is starting to ease some of your concerns about being a diabetic. Yes, it is a big deal and there is much to learn but we don't have to learn it all today. I don't want to get confused here. We are still talking about what to do in the early days after finding out you have diabetes and the idea of thinking long term certainly belongs here. What are we doing right this minute? We are not eating or drinking anything that is high in carbohydrates because we need to bring our blood sugar levels down as soon as possible. What else are we doing? We are beginning to learn more about diabetes and learning more about the foods we can eat and what we should avoid. The other thing that we should be doing now is understanding that nothing happens instantly. Get your head wrapped around the idea that you will make progress in managing your diabetes every day. One could immerse oneself in information and learn all about diabetes relatively quickly and that would be a great thing. However, the more practical approach is more likely to make slow progress with each passing day. The idea that I'm trying to convey here is diabetes is going to be with you for a long time. I think it is more important to commit to making the needed changes and learning how manage it over time rather than trying to figure all of this out right now.

Simply reducing your carbohydrate intake will fix your problem of high blood sugar levels and at this moment, that is the goal. However, eating foods that are low in carbs could also have negative impacts on your health. There are little to no carbs in pepperoni but eating a pile of pepperoni three times a day, every day, is obviously not going to be good for your overall health. For now, reduce the carbs and get those levels down, but as part of your long-term thinking, a balanced diet is the goal.

Exercise is important to regulate blood sugar. You should begin to think about what you can do to increase your activity level and get into better physical shape. Start slow and work your way up to higher goals as you go. Today, you might not even be able to think about exercise. At the time of my diagnosis, I was getting winded trying to do the simplest task and within a few short weeks of reducing my carbohydrate intake, I noticed a profound difference. As soon as you can, start doing something. A short walk will help or if you have steps in your house, when you get to the top, go back down and do it one more time. Make exercise part of your long-term thinking.

6

Conclusion

The goal here was not to answer all the questions you have being newly diagnosed with diabetes but to reduce the anxiety and give some direction about where to start. I hope that I was able to stress that diabetes is a serious disease that you must take seriously to avoid further medical complications. I also hope that I was able to ease your mind in that you now know that this is not a massive mountain that you have to climb. Starting now, reduce your carbohydrate intake and know how many carbs are in everything that you eat and drink. The rest of it is mostly a learning experience that will slowly be built over time. Work closely with and follow the instructions of your healthcare provider and tap into other resources such as reputable websites and content creators on social media. Pay very close attention to the success that you are seeing daily. You should start seeing your numbers improve after a couple of weeks and hopefully even sooner. If for some reason you don't, talk to your doctor and figure out why. If you are struggling with something there is an answer to that problem. The most important thing is that you understand that getting healthy depends on learning how to manage your diabetes and I wish you all the luck in the world as you begin to get healthy.